Addison's Disease

COOKBOOK

Delicious, Easy To Make, Complete Addison's Disease Recipes Guide For Healing Your Body,Reversing Chronic Illness And Healthy Living.

Keen aiden

TABLE OF CONTENTS

CHAPTER ONE

ADDISON'S DISEASE

Addison's disease is a rare but deadly disorder in which the adrenal glands are unable to generate enough of the hormones needed for the body to function normally. These hormones include cortisol, which aids in regulating metabolism and stress response, and aldosterone, which aids in regulating blood pressure and electrolyte balance.

SYMPTOMS

The symptoms of Addison's disease might vary and may progress slowly over time. They may include:

- Weakness and exhaustion: A lack of coordination may result in weakness and weariness, making it difficult to carry out daily activities.
- Weight loss and a decline in appetite: A reduction in appetite may result in weight loss.
- Vomiting and nausea: The digestive system may be affected, resulting in nausea and vomiting.
- Abdominal discomfort: Changes in the digestive system may cause pain in the abdomen.
- Low blood pressure: Addison's disease may result in a drop in blood pressure, which can cause dizziness, weariness, and exhaustion.
- Dimmering of the skin The skin may seem darker or browned as a result of increased producing melanin.

- Muscle and joint pain: A deficiency in cortisol may result in muscle and joint pain.
- Irritability and sadness: The hormonal imbalance may lead to changes in mood, such as irritability and depression.
- A craving for salty foods: A deficiency in aldosterone may result in this craving.

It's neccesary to remember that these symptoms might resemble those of other illnesses, which can make diagnosing Addison's disease challenging. If you are exhibiting any of these symptoms, it is crucial to get a proper diagnosis from your healthcare provider.

CAUSES

The most frequent cause of Addison's disease is autoimmunity-induced destruction of the adrenal glands. The immune system accidentally attacks and destroys the adrenal glands during this process.

Other possible causes of Addison's disease include:

- Infections: Some infections, including tuberculosis, may harm the adrenal glands.
- Cancer: Rarely, cancer may develop in the adrenocortical glands or other parts of the body and result in Addison's disease.
- Genetics: Rarely, a genetic mutation might result in Addison's disease.
- Medications: Some medications, such ketoconazole, may interfere with the generation of cortisol and result in Addison's disease.
- Hemorrhage: Blood loss into the adrenal glands may harm the brain and result in Addison's disease.

It is crucial to remember that the cause of Addison's disease may not always be known. Your healthcare practitioner may order testing if you have been diagnosed with Addison's disease in order to determine the underlying cause and create an effective treatment strategy.

CHAPTER TWO

MANIPULATING ADDISON'S DISEASE

In order to treat Addisonian disease, one must replace the missing hormones with prescription drugs and take precautions to prevent setting off an Addisonian crisis. Here are some crucial steps to managing Addison's disease:

- Hormone replacement therapy: Hormone replacement therapy is the main treatment for Addison's disease. Cortisol and sometimes cocaine are substituted by medications administered as pills or injections. Patients with Addison's disease often need to take these drugs for the rest of their lives.

- Keeping track of hormone levels: Regular hormone level monitoring via blood testing may help ensure that hormone replacement therapy is effective and that hormone levels are within a normal range.

- Managing Strenuous activity may trigger an Addison's disease, therefore it's crucial for patients with the condition to control stress as much as they can. This might include using relaxation techniques, getting enough sleep, and avoiding stressful situations wherever feasible.

- Consuming a balanced diet: Maintaining correct electrolyte balance may be made easier by eating a balanced diet that contains enough salt and fluid consumption.

- Carrying an emergency kit: Patients with Addison's disease should carry an emergency kit that includes a variety of flammable cortisol and instructions on how to use it in the event of an Addisonian crisis.

- Educating others: Patients with Addison's disease should inform family, friends, and coworkers about the illness and how to identify and handle an Addisonian crisis.

Working with health care suppliers: Working together with their healthcare providers can help patients with Addison's disease maintain optimal health and well-being. Regular check-ups, blood tests, and other monitoring may be part of this.

Overall, most persons with Addison's disease may enjoy normal and productive lives with the right diagnosis, treatment, and management.

Diet has a significant role in managing Addison's disease. Here are some dietary recommendations for patients with Addison's disease:

- Appropriate Alt Take: Low levels of aldosterone brought on by Addison's disease may result in low blood pressure and electrolyte imbalances. Elecrolyte balance may be properly maintained by increasing salt intake. To establish the appropriate quantity of salt intake for an individual's requirements, it is crucial to speak with a health care provider or registered dietitian.

- A balanced diet The body may be helped by a balanced diet that contains a range of nutrient-dense foods in order to get the nutrients it needs to sustain optimal health. This may consist of a variety of fruits, vegetables, whole grains, clean proteins, and healthy fats.

- Refraining from high-potassium foods: Patients with Addison's disease may struggle to control their blood sugar levels, so it's crucial to stay away from foods rich in sugar, such bananas, tomatoes, and pears.

- Consuming frequent little meals: Eating often little meals throughout the day may help maintain stable blood sugar levels and prevent hypoglycemic symptoms.

- Adequate fluid intake: Adequate fluid intake may help maintain proper hydration and electrolyte balance.

- Avoiding caffeine and alcohol: These substances may affect the development of the cardiovascular system and exacerbate Addison's disease symptoms.

Patients with Addison's disease must collaborate closely with their healthcare physician and a certified dietitian to create a personalized dietary plan that addresses their unique requirements.

CHAPTER 3

MENU PLAN

Here is an example menu plan for a person with Addison's disease:

BREAKFAST:

- Scrambled eggs with bacon and muffaletta
- Whole wheat toast
- Orange juice

SNACK:

- Apple is sliced with almond butter.

LUNCH:

- Grilled chicken breakfast
- Quinoa salad with tomatoes, cucumbers, andfeta cheese
- Vinaigrette dressing with lemon

SNACK:

- Greek yogurt with a variety of fruit and honey

DINNER

- baked samon with lemon and herbs.
- Baked sweet potatoes
- Stewed Bologna

CHAPTER FOUR

ADDISON DISEASE DIET RECIPES

PEANUT BUTTER BANANA OAT COOKIES

INGREDIENTS:

- 1 cup rolled oats
- 1 ripe banana, mashed
- 1/2 cup natural peanut butter
- 1/4 cup honey
- 1 tsp vanilla extract
- 1/4 tsp salt

INSTRUCTIONS:

1. Preheat the oven to 350°F and line a baking sheet with parchment paper.
2. In a large bowl, mix together the oats, mashed banana, peanut butter, honey, vanilla extract, and salt until fully combined.

3. Drop spoonfuls of the mixture onto the prepared baking sheet and flatten slightly with a fork.

4. Bake for 10-12 minutes or until golden brown.

GREEK YOGURT PARFAIT

INGREDIENTS:

- 1 cup plain Greek yogurt
- 1/2 cup mixed berries (strawberries, blueberries, raspberries, etc.)
- 1/4 cup chopped nuts (almonds, walnuts, etc.)
- 1 tbsp honey

INSTRUCTIONS:

1. In a small bowl, mix together the Greek yogurt and honey.

2. In a parfait glass or bowl, layer the yogurt mixture, mixed berries, and chopped nuts.

3. Repeat the layers until all the ingredients are used up.

4. Serve immediately.

CHOCOLATE CHIA PUDDING

INGREDIENTS:

- 1/2 cup chia seeds
- 2 cups unsweetened almond milk
- 1/4 cup unsweetened cocoa powder
- 1/4 cup honey
- 1 tsp vanilla extract

INSTRUCTIONS:

1. In a large bowl, whisk together the chia seeds, almond milk, cocoa powder, honey, and vanilla extract until fully combined.

2. Cover the bowl and refrigerate for at least 2 hours or overnight, until the mixture has thickened into a pudding-like consistency.

3. Serve in bowls.

CINNAMON APPLE CHIPS

INGREDIENTS:

- 2 apples, thinly sliced
- 1 tbsp cinnamon
- 1 tbsp honey

INSTRUCTIONS:

1. Preheat the oven to 225°F and line a baking sheet with parchment paper.
2. In a small bowl, mix together the cinnamon and honey.
3. Brush the apple slices with the cinnamon and honey mixture and arrange them in a single layer on the prepared
4. Bake for 1-2 hours or until the apple slices are crisp and golden brown.
5. Serve as a snack or dessert.

BLUEBERRY CRISP

INGREDIENTS:

- 2 cups fresh or frozen blueberries

- 1/2 cup rolled oats
- 1/4 cup almond flour
- 1/4 cup chopped nuts (almonds, walnuts, etc.)
- 1/4 cup honey
- 1 tsp cinnamon
- 1/4 tsp salt
- 2 tbsp coconut oil

INSTRUCTIONS:

1. Preheat the oven to 350°F and lightly grease a baking dish.
2. In a large bowl, mix together the blueberries, rolled oats, almond flour, chopped nuts, honey, cinnamon, and salt until fully combined.
3. Pour the mixture into the prepared baking dish and dot with small pieces of coconut oil.
4. Bake for 30-35 minutes or until the top is golden brown and the blueberries are bubbling.

5. Serve warm with a dollop of Greek yogurt or whipped cream, if desired.

ONE SKILLET TUSCAN CHICKEN

INGREDIENTS

- 1 lb boneless, skinless chicken breasts, cubed
- 8 oz mushrooms, sliced
- 1/2 yellow onion, diced
- 2-3 cloves garlic, minced
- 2 medium tomatoes, diced
- 1 15 oz can Cannellini Beans, drained and rinsed
- 1/2 cup chopped sun-dried tomatoes
- 1/3 cup black pitted olives
- 2-3 Tablespoon extra virgin olive oil
- 1 Tablespoon honey
- 1 Tablespoon balsamic vinegar
- 1 teaspoon oregano
- 1 teaspoon thyme

• 2 Tablespoon fresh basil, chopped for garnish

• Salt & pepper to taste

INSTRUCTIONS

1. In a large skillet heat oil over medium heat, add the cubed chicken pieces and cook for about 8 minutes on both sides, until cooked through. Remove chicken and transfer to a plate.

2. Add 1 Tbsp of olive oil to the skillet and sauté the sliced mushrooms 5 – 7 minutes until the mushrooms are tender and the juices have evaporated. Set aside.

3. Add another 1 Tbsp olive oil to the skillet and the diced onion. Sauté the onions 3 – 4 minutes until translucent. Add the minced garlic to the onions and sauté together one more minute. Add salt and pepper to taste while cooking.

4. Add 1 Tbsp olive oil to the skillet and toss the diced tomatoes, sun-dried tomatoes,

Cannellini beans, and black olives. Season again with salt and freshly ground black pepper. Sprinkle in the oregano, thyme and drizzle the balsamic vinegar and honey. Stir a few minutes.

5. Next, add the cooked chicken and mushrooms to the skillet – stir and cook 1-2 minutes, or until chicken is heated through. Add more salt and pepper if needed.

6. Serve hot, garnished with the fresh basil.

CHICKEN NOODLE CASSEROLE

INGREDIENTS

- 2 cups uncooked egg noodles
- 2 cups cooked shredded chicken
- 1 package (10 ounces) frozen peas and carrots, thawed
- 1 package (10 ounces) frozen corn, thawed
- 1 cup milk
- 1 can (10 ounces) cream of chicken soup
- 1 can (10 ounces) cream of mushroom soup

- salt and pepper to taste
- 1/2 Tablespoon dried minced onion
- 2 Tablespoons melted butter
- 1/2 teaspoon garlic powder
- 1/2 teaspoon Italian seasoning

INSTRUCTIONS

1. Preheat oven to 375° F. Spray a 9x13 inch baking dish with nonstick spray.
2. Boil egg noodles according to package directions. Drain water.
3. Meanwhile, in a large bowl combine all the other remaining ingredients. Add cooked noodles to mixture. Gently stir to combine everything. Pour into prepared baking dish. Cover with foil.
4. Bake 30 minutes or until heated through. Remove from oven and let stand 5 minutes before serving. Enjoy!

ITALIAN CHICKEN AND ORZO

INGREDIENTS

- 2 chicken breasts chopped into bite size (approx.1 pound)
- 1 tablespoon olive oil
- 3 tablespoons pesto, divided
- 1/2 onion, chopped
- 1 cup sliced carrots
- 1 cup zucchini, quartered
- 1 red bell pepper, chopped
- 1 cup uncooked orzo
- 2 garlic cloves, minced
- 1 14.5 oz. can crushed tomatoes
- 2 cups low sodium chicken broth
- 1 teaspoon chicken bouillon, optional*
- 1/2 teaspoon dried oregano
- 1/4 teaspoon salt *
- 1/4 teaspoon pepper
- 1/4 teaspoon red pepper flakes
- 1/2 cup freshly grated Parmesan cheese

Garnish (Optional)

- freshly grated Parmesan cheese
- fresh parsley

INSTRUCTIONS

1. Heat olive oil in a large NONSTICK pan over medium high heat until very hot. Toss chicken with 1 tablespoon pesto and add to pan along with onions, carrots and zucchini. Sauté for three minutes then add red bell pepper, orzo and garlic and cook an additional 2 minutes.

2. Stir in crushed tomatoes, 2 tablespoons pesto, chicken broth, chicken bouillon and seasonings. Bring to a simmer, cover and reduce heat to medium low. Simmer for 8-12 minutes, or until vegetables and orzo are tender, stirring every 5 minutes so the orzo doesn't burn, covering pot after each stir.

3. Stir in Parmesan cheese. Taste and season with additional salt and pepper if desired. Garnish with fresh Parmesan and parsley (optional).

CHICKEN SALAD SANDWICHES

INGREDIENTS

- 1 1/2cups chopped cooked chicken or turkey
- 1medium stalk celery, chopped (1/2 cup)
- 1small onion, finely chopped (1/3 cup)
- 1/2cup mayonnaise or salad dressing
- 1/4teaspoon salt
- 1/4teaspoon pepper
- 8slices bread

INSTRUCTIONS

1. In medium bowl, mix all ingredients except bread.
2. Spread mixture on 4 bread slices.
3. Top with remaining bread.

EASY ROTISSERIE CHICKEN TACOS

INGREDIENTS

- 2 cups salsa (see our homemade recipe here, or use your favorite jarred salsa)
- 1 cup water
- 2 tablespoons tomato paste
- ½ teaspoon coriander
- 1 teaspoon chili powder
- 1 teaspoon ground cumin
- 1 small rotisserie chicken, meat removed from the bones (you'll want about 1½ pounds of picked chicken meat)
- 6 tablespoons vegetable oil
- 12 white or yellow 6" corn tortillas
- 8 ounces pepper jack cheese, shredded
- 4 cups shredded iceberg lettuce
- 8 ounces Monterey jack cheese, shredded

Toppings

- Sliced black olives

- Sliced pickled jalapenos
- Thinly sliced red onion
- Avocado wedges
- Sour cream
- Lime juice
- Fresh cilantro

INSTRUCTIONS

1. Preheat the oven to 450 degrees F.
2. Have a roasting pan with high sides ready that can hold 12 completed folded tacos (or 2 pans with 6 each).
3. In a large skillet, place salsa, water and tomato paste. Start burner on medium, stir and combine.
4. Add the coriander, chili powder and cumin and stir again.
5. Shred the cooked chicken pieces into the salsa mixture and heat to hot then hold to keep warm.

6. Brush two sheet pans with half of the oil. Lay out the corn tortillas, 6 per tray and brush the tops with the other half of the oil.

7. Divide the pepper jack between the 12 tortillas.

8. Divide the warm chicken mixture between the 12 tortillas, on top of the pepper jack but not completely to the edges.

9. Place in the oven for 12-15 minutes or until the edges start to get a little crispy and the mixture is hot and bubbly. Rotate pans half way through for even browning.

10. Remove one pan at a time from the oven and quickly top with half the lettuce. Then pick up each tortilla, fold in half and place in the reserved dish or pan, letting each taco stay folded by leaning on the one next to it, or the side of the pan. They will stay in this shape once folded hot. Repeat for the second pan. Turn off oven. (Note: Tacos are hot so we suggest that you use tongs to remove and fold.)

11. Then take the 12 folded tacos and top with the Monterey jack cheese and place back in the oven with the oven off for 4-5 minutes. The residual heat will melt the jack cheese over the lettuce.

12. Serve hot with whatever toppings you want including sliced back olives, pickled jalapenos, thinly sliced red onion, avocado wedges, sour cream, lime juice, fresh cilantro, etc.

ITALIAN CHICKEN

INGREDIENTS

For the chicken:

- 1 cup all-purpose flour
- 2 teaspoon kosher salt
- 1 ½ teaspoon black pepper
- 2 teaspoon Italian seasoning
- 1 Tablespoon powdered sugar
- 6 boneless, skinless chicken breasts
- 1 cup whole milk

- 1 teaspoon lemon juice
- 3 Tablespoon olive oil

For the sauce:

- 2 Tablespoon olive oil
- 4 cloves garlic, minced
- ¼ cup sun dried tomatoes in oil, drained and finely diced
- 3 Tablespoon cornstarch, divided
- 1 cup chicken broth
- 3 cups fresh spinach, roughly chopped
- 1 cup heavy cream
- 1 cup whole milk
- 1 teaspoon kosher salt
- ½ teaspoon pepper (don't skimp on this)
- 1 cup parmesan cheese, grated
- 1 box (16oz) linguine noodles

INSTRUCTIONS

1. Place raw chicken breast into a bowl and pour milk and lemon juice over the top. Cover and refrigerate for 2-4 hours. You can

also do this in the morning, so that it's ready at dinner time!

2. When ready to cook, create your chicken crust. In a pie plate, or shallow dish, combine flour, salt, pepper, Italian seasoning, and powdered sugar.

3. Drain chicken from milk marinade and dip into the flour, coating evenly.

4. Heat a large skillet with olive oil over medium high heat. Place chicken strips in hot skillet for about 3 minutes on each side. Remove and place onto a foil lined baking sheet.

5. Bake chicken in 350 degree oven for about 18-20 minutes.

6. While the chicken bakes, cook your linguine (or favorite pasta) according to package.

7. To make the sauce, using the same skillet as the chicken, add additional olive oil, scraping the bits from the pan. Over medium heat, add garlic and sun dried tomatoes to the pan, heat for several minutes.

8. Sprinkle 1 Tbsp cornstarch over the tomatoes, and mix thoroughly.

9. Add chicken broth, whisk until combined. Cook for about 5 minutes.

10. In a small bowl, mix remaining cornstarch with milk and whisk. Add to the broth and continue whisking while adding in the cream, spinach, salt, and pepper.

11. Turn heat to low and simmer until sauce thickens and spinach wilts. Add in parmesan cheese.

12. Stir and heat on low until chicken and noodles are done.

13. Serve in a large bowl and enjoy.

BETTER-THAN-TAKEOUT CASHEW CHICKEN

INGREDIENTS

Stir-Fry:

- 3 tablespoons cornstarch
- 1/2 teaspoon salt

- 1/2 teaspoon pepper
- about 1.25 pounds boneless skinless chicken breasts, diced into 1-inch pieces
- 2 tablespoons sesame oil
- 1 tablespoon olive oil
- 2 heaping cups broccoli florets
- 1 cup red bell peppers, diced small
- 1 cup shelled frozen edamame
- 2 cloves garlic, finely minced or pressed
- 1 cup unsalted dry-roasted whole cashews
- 3/4 to 1 cup green onions, sliced into thin rounds (from about 3 or 4 green onions)

Sauce:

- 3 tablespoons low-sodium soy sauce
- 2 tablespoons honey, or to taste
- 1 tablespoon rice wine vinegar
- 1 tablespoon Asian chili garlic sauce
- 3/4 teaspoon ground ginger

INSTRUCTIONS

1. To a gallon-sized ziptop bag, add the cornstarch, salt, pepper, chicken, seal, and shake to coat chicken evenly.

2. To a large skillet, add the oils, chicken, and cook for about 4 to 5 minutes over medium-high heat, flipping and stirring so all sides cook evenly. Chicken should be about 80-90% cooked through.

3. Add the broccoli, bell peppers, edamame , garlic, and stir to combine. Cook for about 3 to 4 minutes or until vegetables are crisp-tender and chicken is cooked through; stir intermittently. While vegetables cook, make the sauce.

4. To a medium bowl add the soy sauce, honey, rice wine vinegar, chili-garlic sauce, ginger, and whisk to combine; set aside.

5. Add the cashews to the skillet and stir to combine.

6. Add the sauce and stir to combine. Allow sauce to simmer over medium-low heat for 1 to 2 minutes.

7. Add the green onions, stir to combine, and serve immediately.

CHICKEN AND STUFFING CASSEROLE

INGREDIENTS

- 10.5 oz can cream of chicken and mushroom soup or use cream of chicken soup
- 10.5 oz can cream of celery soup
- 1 cup whole milk
- 3 cup cooked chicken breast diced
- 1/2 cup salted butter divided
- 1 cup yellow onion diced
- 1 cup celery diced
- 3 cloves garlic minced
- 1 1/2 cup water
- 6 oz package Stovetop stuffing chicken flavor
- salt and pepper to taste

INSTRUCTIONS

1. Preheat oven to 350 degrees F.

2. In a large bowl whisk together both cans of soup and the milk.

3. Add cooked chicken to the soup mixture and stir to combine.

4. Spread chicken and soup mixture in a 3 quart casserole dish, or a 9×13 baking dish.

5. Sprinkle with black pepper and just a dash of salt, if needed. Set aside.

6. In a 12 inch skillet combine 4 tablespoons butter, onions, celery, and minced garlic over medium heat. Saute until the onions and celery are soft and translucent.

7. Add the entire contents of the stuffing package to the skillet.Pour water over the stuffing and stir to mix everything together.

8. Spread stuffing mixture over the chicken soup mixture in the casserole dish.

9. Melt remaining 4 tablespoons of butter and drizzle over the top of the stuffing.

10. Bake casserole, uncovered, in the oven for approximately 30 minutes or until the stuffing is browned and the soup mixture is hot and bubbly.
11. Serve immediately.

CHICKEN BACON RANCH CASSEROLE

INGREDIENTS

- 12 slices of bacon cooked and chopped (divided)
- 6 cups of penne pasta about 4 cups dry, cooked and drained
- 3 or 4 boneless skinless chicken breasts (about 2 pounds), cut into bite-size pieces
- 1 ½ teaspoon of salt divided
- ½ teaspoon of pepper
- 3 tablespoons Ranch seasoning mix divided
- 8 tablespoons 1 stick of butter (divided)
- 2 tablespoons of olive oil divided
- ⅔ cup onion chopped
- 2 teaspoons of minced garlic

- ½ cup flour
- 1 teaspoon Italian seasoning
- 1 teaspoon dried basil
- 3 cups of chicken broth
- 1 cup of heavy cream
- ½ cup shaved parmesan cheese
- ¼ cup sun-dried tomatoes patted dry if oil-packed and chopped
- 3 cups of Italian style cheese
- ¼ cup of chopped fresh parsley or 2 teaspoons of dried parsley this is optional

INSTRUCTIONS

1. Preheat oven to 350°. Grease 9×13 inch pan
2. In a medium bowl, combine chicken with ½ teaspoon salt, ½ teaspoon pepper, and 2 tablespoons Ranch dressing mix
3. In a large skillet over medium high heat, melt 2 tablespoons butter and 1 tablespoon olive oil.

4. Add a single layer of chicken. Cook until golden on each side, about 4 to 5 minutes per side. Remove with a slotted spoon.

5. Repeat with the remaining chicken, using 2 more tablespoons butter and the remaining 1 tablespoon olive oil.

6. Reduce heat to medium. Saute onion in pan drippings until soft. Add garlic and saute for 1 more minute.

7. To the same pan (with the onion and garlic), add 3 tablespoons butter. When butter is melted, add flour, Italian seasoning, basil, remaining 1 teaspoon salt, and remaining 1 tablespoon Ranch dressing mix. Stir.

8. Using a whisk, gradually add chicken broth (¼ to ½ cup at a time), stirring to combine well with the flour mixture.

9. Add heavy cream. Continue to stir, heating until bubbly.

10. Add parmesan and stir until cheese is melted. Remove from heat.

11. To the sauce, add 8 slices of chopped bacon, sun-dried tomatoes, chicken, and pasta.

12. Combine the pasta with the sauce.

13. Pour pasta mixture into a greased 9×13 pan.

14. Sprinkle with the remaining 4 pieces of chopped bacon. Top with Italian cheese. Sprinkle with dried or fresh chopped parsley, if desired.

15. Bake uncovered at 350° for 20 minutes or until cheese is melted and edges are bubbly.

CHICKEN ALFREDO BAKE

INGREDIENTS

- 16 ounces penne pasta
- 5 tablespoons salted butter
- 4 ounces cream cheese
- 1 tablespoon garlic, minced
- 1 tablespoon garlic powder
- 1 tablespoon onion powder
- 1 tablespoon Italian seasoning
- 1 teaspoon black pepper

- 1 tablespoon flour
- 2 cups heavy whipping cream
- 1 cup whole milk
- 2 cups mozzarella cheese shredded, divided
- 1½ cups parmesan cheese shredded, divided
- 2 cups chicken breast shredded or chopped

INSTRUCTIONS

1. Preheat oven to 350°F.
2. Prepare pasta to al dente and set aside.
3. In a Dutch oven, melt butter over medium heat. Add cream cheese. Use a whisk to stir.
4. Add minced garlic, garlic powder, onion powder, black pepper, and Italian seasoning. Whisk until mixed and butter/cream cheese are melted.
5. Add flour and mix well.
6. Add heavy whipping cream one cup at a time, continue to stir. Add milk.
7. Add one cup of mozzarella cheese and one cup of parmesan cheese, stir to mix and melt.

8. Once all the sauce is melted, stir in chicken and pasta.

9. Pour in 9×13 pan that has been sprayed with nonstick spray.

10. Top with remaining one cup of mozzarella and ½ cup of parmesan cheese.

11. Bake for 10 to 15 minutes to melt the cheese. Turn on the broiler for a couple of minutes to brown.

CHICKEN RICE CASSEROLE

INGREDIENTS

- 1 lb. Boneless, skinless chicken thighs
- 1 cup Basmati rice
- 3 tbsp. Olive oil
- 1 medium Onion, diced
- 2 medium Carrots, shredded
- 2 cups Chicken broth
- 1 tsp. Favorite Chicken Seasoning* (or to taste)
- 1 tsp. Salt and pepper, to taste** (or to taste)

- ¼ tsp. turmeric, optional (for color)***

INSTRUCTIONS

1. Preheat the oven to 450 °F.
2. In a large skillet, sauté the chopped onion with olive oil over medium-high heat for about 3 minutes. Add the carrots and cook for another 3 minutes.
3. Add the chicken and season it with salt, pepper, and your favorite chicken seasoning.
4. Cook the chicken for 5-7 minutes.
5. Transfer the chicken to a medium casserole dish and add the rice and chicken broth. Stir well.
6. Cover the casserole with foil and bake for 40 minutes.

QUICK & EASY CHICKEN FLAUTAS

INGREDIENTS

- 2 cans (12.5 oz each) chicken drained & flaked

- 6 oz cream cheese softened
- ⅓ cup salsa
- 1 cup shredded cheese any variety
- ¼ teaspoon cumin
- ¼ teaspoon garlic powder
- ¼ teaspoon onion powder
- ¼ teaspoon chili powder
- 12 8" flour tortillas

INSTRUCTIONS

1. Heat oven to 400°. Prepare a cookie sheet by lining with parchment paper or tin foil, or you can spray the pan with cooking spray.

2. Combine drained and flaked chicken, cream cheese, salsa, cheese, cumin, garlic powder, onion powder, and chili powder into a mixing bowl. Stir together until well combined.

3. Spread 3 tablespoons (a large spoonful) of chicken mixture onto a tortilla. Roll up tightly and place seam side down on a

cookie sheet. Repeat with remaining tortillas. .

4. Spray the tops of the flautas with cooking spray. Don't soak them but you want them to have a decent coating of cooking spray so they will get really brown and crispy.

5. Bake for 18-20 minutes or until they reach desired crispness that you want. Let cool for about 5-10 minutes before serving so the filling can cool and come together.

1. Serve with dips of your choice (sour cream, salsa, guacamole).

OLD FASHIONED GOULASH

INGREDIENTS

- 2 pounds lean ground beef
- 2 large yellow onions, chopped
- 4 cloves garlic, chopped
- 2 cups water
- 1 cup beef broth
- Two 15-ounce cans tomato sauce

- Two 15-ounce cans diced tomatoes
- 1 tablespoon Italian seasoning
- 1 tablespoon oregano
- 3 bay leaves
- 2 tablespoons Worcestershire sauce
- ½ teaspoon salt
- ½ teaspoon garlic powder
- ½ teaspoon pepper
- 2 cups elbow macaroni, uncooked
- 1 cup shredded cheddar cheese

INSTRUCTIONS

1. In a Dutch oven, saute the ground beef over medium-high heat, until no pink remains. Break up meat while sauteing; spoon off any grease.

2. Add the onions to the pot and saute until they are tender about 5 minutes. Add 2 cups water and one cup beef broth, along with the tomato sauce, tomatoes, garlic, bay leaves, Worcestershire sauce and seasonings. Stir

well. Place a lid on the pot and allow this to cook for 20 to 25 minutes.

3. Add the elbow macaroni, stir well, return the lid to the pot and simmer until pasta is al dente, about 4-5 minutes. Pasta will cook a bit more when you remove from heat. IMPORTANT: be careful not to cook your pasta too long, mushy goulash is not good!

4. Remove from heat, remove the bay leaves. Serve warm and top with shredded cheddar cheese.

ROTISSERIE CHICKEN SKILLET

INGREDIENTS

- 1 whole rotisserie chicken, or 3 1/2 cups cooked chicken meat
- 1/2 cup uncooked orzo pasta
- 2 tablespoons olive or vegetable oil
- 2 cups carrots cut on the bias
- 1 cup onion cut into thick strips
- 2 cups chicken stock

- 1/2 teaspoon garlic powder
- 1 teaspoon kosher salt
- 1/2 teaspoon freshly ground black pepper
- 1/2 cup chopped fresh parsley
- 1 cup frozen peas
- 1/2 cup heavy cream
- 1/2 cup freshly grated Parmesan cheese

INSTRUCTIONS

1. Pick the meat from the cooked chicken and roughly cut up and set aside.
2. In a large dry skillet pan over medium high heat, cook orzo until lightly browned; about 3 minutes stirring frequently.
3. Remove browned orzo to a bowl and add oil to hot pan.
4. Add carrots and onion and sauté for 4 minutes.
5. Add orzo back in along with stock, garlic powder, salt and pepper. Cover and reduce heat to a medium simmer and simmer to cook the orzo, about 8-10 minutes.

6. Uncover and add parsley, peas, and cream along with cooked chicken.
7. Increase heat and cook just to bring the dish to temperature and incorporate the ingredients.
8. Serve with grated Parmesan sprinkled over the top.

ONE PAN ITALIAN CHICKEN SKILLET RECIPE

INGREDIENTS

- 1 pound chicken breast, cut into bite sized pieces
- 2 Tbsp extra virgin olive oil, avocado oil, or unrefined coconut oil
- 4 fresh garlic cloves, minced
- 8 oz fresh button mushrooms
- 2 red bell pepper, chopped
- 1 bunch asparagus, ends trimmed and cut in halves

- 1 medium zucchini, sliced
- 1 Tbsp dry Italian seasoning
- 2 Tbsps high quality balsamic vinegar
- sea salt and black pepper, to your taste

INSTRUCTIONS

1. Heat oil over med-high heat in a large skillet.
2. Add mushrooms and garlic, and saute for 5 minutes.
3. Then, add chicken and cook for another 5 minutes until browned.
4. Add Italian seasoning, balsamic vinegar and season with salt and pepper to your taste.
5. Add in bell pepper, asparagus and zucchini, and cook for an additional 10 minutes or until veggies are tender and everything is cooked through.

ONE POT CHEESY CHICKEN BROCCOLI RICE

INGREDIENTS

- 2 tablespoons olive oil
- 3 boneless, skinless chicken breasts (cut into small, bite-sized pieces)
- 1 teaspoon salt
- ½ teaspoon pepper
- 1 cup uncooked basmati rice OR long-grain rice
- 2 ½ cups chicken broth
- 1 bag (12 oz) frozen steamable broccoli (about 2 cups chopped broccoli)
- 2 cups shredded cheddar cheese

INSTRUCTIONS

1. In a 12-inch skillet pan (make sure it has a lid) over medium-high heat, add the olive oil, chicken, salt, and pepper.

1. Cook 4-6 minutes, stirring frequently, until chicken is mostly non-pink in the middle. Chicken should be white on the outside.

2. Drain the excess liquid and oil from the chicken.

3. Add rice and chicken broth. Bring to a boil. Once boiling, cover with lid, and reduce heat to medium-low.

4. Simmer for 15 minutes or until water is absorbed and rice is cooked.

2. While rice and chicken is simmering, cook the microwaveable broccoli in the microwave following the instructions on package.

5. Once done, chop up the broccoli into smaller pieces, if wanted.

3. When rice is done cooking, add broccoli and 1 cup of the cheese into the skillet pan. Stir together.

6. Top with the remaining 1 cup shredded cheese and cover with the lid. Let cook for

about 2 more minutes or until cheese is melted.

4. Serve immediately.

ONE PAN GREEK LEMON CHICKEN AND RICE

INGREDIENTS

Marinade

- •2 tsp dried oregano
- •1 tsp dried minced onion
- •4-5 cloves garlic, minced
- •zest of 1 lemon
- •1/2 tsp kosher salt
- •1/2 tsp black pepper
- •1-2 Tbsp olive oil to make a loose paste
- •5 bone-in, skin on chicken thighs

Rice

- •1 1/2 Tbsp olive oil
- •1 large yellow onion, peeled and diced

- •1 cup dry long-grain white rice (NOT minute or quick cooking varieties)
- •2 cups chicken stock
- •1 1/4 tsp dried oregano
- •5 cloves garlic, minced
- •3/4 tsp kosher salt
- •1/2 tsp black pepper
- •lemon slices, optional
- •fresh minced parsley, for garnish
- •extra lemon zest, for garnish

INSTRUCTIONS

1. In a large resealable plastic bag, add all marinade ingredients (except chicken), and massage to combine. Add chicken thighs and turn/massage to coat. Refrigerate 15 minutes up to overnight.
2. Preheat oven to 350 F degrees.
3. Add 1 1/2 Tbsp olive oil to large cast iron or heavy oven safe skillet, and heat over MED-HIGH heat. Shake off excess marinade from chicken thighs and add chicken thighs,

skin side down, to pan. Cook 4-5 minutes per side. Remove to plate and wipe skillet lightly with a paper towel to remove any blackened bits, reserving chicken grease in pan.

4. Reduce heat to MED and add onion to pan. Cook 3-4 minutes, until softened and slightly charred. Add garlic and cook 1 minute. Add rice, oregano, salt and pepper. Stir together and cook 1 minute.

5. Pour in chicken stock, raise temperature to MED-HIGH and bring to a simmer. Once simmering, nestle chicken thighs on top of the rice mixture.

6. Cover with lid or foil, and bake 35 minutes. Uncover, return to oven and bake an additional 10-15 minutes, until liquid is removed, rice is tender, and chicken is cooked through.

7. Garnish as desired and serve.

LOWER CARB STRAWBERRY SMOOTHIE

INGREDIENTS

- 5 medium strawberry
- 1 cup unsweetened soy milk (or unsweetened almond milk)
- 1/2 cup low-fat Greek-style yogurt
- 6 ice cubes

INSTRUCTIONS

1. Place all ingredients in a blender and blend until smooth.
2. Pour into a glass and garnish with a strawberry.

EASY TIGERNUT BUTTER RECIPE (NUT FREE & PALEO)

INGREDIENTS

- •1 cup tigernut flour
- •1/4 cup coconut oil

INSTRUCTIONS

1. First, add tigernut flour and coconut oil to a food processor.
2. Process on high for 1 minute. Then, use a rubber spatula or spoon to scrape down the sides of the food processor.
3. Then, process for another minute. Continue processing until smooth and creamy.
4. Finally, store tigernut butter in a Mason jar or jar with lid.

KETO TRIPLE BERRY SMOOTHIE

INGREDIENTS

- 1/2 cup coconut milk
- 1.5 cups unsweetened almond milk
- 2/3 cup frozen raspberries
- 2/3 cup strawberries
- 1/2 cup blackberries
- 1 tbsp sugar-free whipped cream optional
- Other optional add ins: low-carb sweetener, collagen powder, protein powder, nut butter, MCT oil

INSTRUCTIONS

1. Place everything in a blender and process until smooth. If it's too thick add more coconut or almond milk, if it's too thin for your liking add in some ice and a little xanthan gum to thicken.
2. Top with optional whipped cream if desired.

HEALTHY FRENCH TOAST FOR A CLEAN EATING PLAN

INGREDIENTS

- ½ cup egg whites
- ½ cup milk (for non-dairy, unsweetened almond or rice work best)
- 1 tsp. ground cinnamon
- 1 tsp. pure vanilla extract
- 6 slices whole grain bread (no sugar added)
- maple syrup or honey for topping

INSTRUCTIONS

1. Combine your egg whites, milk, cinnamon and vanilla in a bowl. Whisk until well blended.
2. Soak your bread in the mixture, one slice at a time, until it's partially saturated (Don't let it get too soggy or it will be a drag to get it out of the bowl) Make sure you soak on both sides of each slice.

3. To keep things lower in fat, cook in a non-stick pan without any oil.

4. Keep the heat low to medium low so it doesn't burn. Cook a bit longer than you would regular french toast to be sure the egg gets cooked at the lower temperature.

5. Plate your food and top with your favorite French toast toppings!

EASY GLUTEN-FREE FOCACCIA RECIPE

INGREDIENTS

Wet Ingredients

- 1 tbsp Sugar
- 2 tbsp Olive oil
- 2 1/4 tsp Active Dry Yeast
- 2 1/4 cup Warm Water

Dry Ingredients

- 3 cup Gluten Free All Purpose 1:1 Flour Blend

- 1/2 cup Almond Flour
- 2 tsp Baking Powder

Focaccia Toppings

- 2 tbsp Olive Oil
- 1/2 cup Pitted Olives
- 2 tbsp Rosemary, chopped
- 1 tsp Garlic Powder
- 1/4 tsp Sea Salt

INSTRUCTIONS

1. Whisk together gluten-free all purpose flour, almond flour, baking powder, and salt in a large bowl and set aside.

2. Add the warm water (120°-130°F), active dry yeast, sugar, and olive oil into a small bowl and stir to combine. Set the mixture aside for at least 15 minutes, or until the yeast blooms, or appears to have foam on the top.

3. Add the yeast mixture into the large bowl with the flour. Mix well until thoroughly

combined. You will notice that the dough is closer to batter in appearance. This is completely okay! No need to worry or knead the dough!

4. Using a clean towel or plastic wrap, cover the bowl, and set it aside to rise. Try to keep the dough in a warm place. Let the dough rise for at least an hour. You will notice that the dough has doubled in size.

5. Drizzle 1 tbsp of olive oil onto a baking sheet and spread evenly. Pour the dough onto the prepared baking sheet. Spread the dough into a rectangular shape until it is spread evenly. The size should be about 8 X 11" and ¾ inches thick.

6. Add your toppings to the dough. If you are using pitted olives, gently press the olives into the dough. Sprinkle rosemary and garlic onto the dough. (If you want to press dimples into the focaccia, do so with lightly oiled fingers right before it goes into the oven.)

7. Set the dough aside and let it rest one final time for 30 minutes. During this time, preheat the oven to 400°F.

8. Remove the cover from the dough. Drizzle 2 tbsp olive oil onto the focaccia dough. Transfer to the oven and bake for 25-30 minutes or until golden brown.

9. Remove the dough from the oven. Let it cool for about 5 minutes. Top with sea salt and cut into squares. Serve & Enjoy!

EASY HOMEMADE BERRY YOGURT

INGREDIENTS

- 4 3/4 cups milk at room temperature (do not use fat free milk, it does not work well)
- 8 ounces of high quality plain yogurt (yes this is more than most recipes, but it works)
- 10 tablespoons of powdered milk
- For flavored yogurt use:
- 1/4 cup of jelly or jam, I use homemade (we like jelly because it has no seeds in it and we

like the berry flavors best because they have a stronger flavor)

INSTRUCTIONS

1. Your milk must be at room temperature! .

2. Once the milk is at room temperature mix together the remaining ingredients, including the jelly. I find this mixes together best in a blender. It helps the jelly mix in really well. But if you are just making plain yogurt you can mix together with a whisk.

3. Fill yogurt cups and heat in yogurt maker for 7-8 hours.

4. Remove, let cool to room temperature, refrigerate, and enjoy.

JOLLY GREEN GOODNESS SMOOTHIE

INGREDIENTS

- 1 cup almond milk or milk of choice
- 1 cup spinach or leafy greens of choice
- 1/2 medium pear or apple

- 1/2 cucumber
- zest and juice of one lemon
- 1/2 inch ginger root or pinch of ground ginger optional
- 1 cup ice optional

Optional add-ins (not all together!)*:

- 1 tablespoon almond butter or other nut butter of choice
- 1 date
- 1 teaspoon flax/hemp/chia seeds
- 1 tablespoon unsweetened coconut
- 1/2 cup frozen cauliflower frozen, this is a great sub for ice, to maintain a creamy texture while adding more nutrients
- 1/2 cup zucchini diced

INSTRUCTIONS

1. This could not be any simpler…add everything to a blender, mix and enjoy!

SAUTEED ASPARAGUS WITH LEMON

INGREDIENTS

- 1 Land O' Lakes Savory Butter and Olive Oil Saute Express Cube
- 1 bunch fresh asparagus
- 1/2 lemon thinly sliced - optional

INSTRUCTIONS

1. Place saute express cube into skillet and melt over low heat.
2. Add asparagus, increase heat to medium and toss until coated.
3. Cook for approximately 5 minutes until asparagus is tender. If you're substituting larger asparagus it will take longer to cook.
4. Garnish with lemon slices if desired.

SUN-DRIED TOMATO CHICKEN PASTA

INGREDIENTS

Chicken

- 2 medium chicken breasts (approx. 1 pound) sliced horizontally through the equator, pounded to an even thickness
- 2 1/2 tablespoons oil from sun-dried tomatoes divided
- 1/2 tsp EACH garlic powder, onion powder, paprika
- 1/4 tsp EACH salt, pepper

Pasta

- 1 lb. cellentani or pasta of choice
- 1 tablespoon oil from sun-dried tomatoes jar
- 2 tablespoons unsalted butter
- 1 large shallot chopped (about ½ cup)
- 4 oz. sun-dried tomatoes in oil rinsed, chopped into strips (1 heaping cup)
- 4 garlic cloves minced

- 1/4 teaspoon red pepper flakes
- 3 tablespoons all-purpose flour
- 1 1/2 cups low sodium chicken broth
- 1 cup milk
- 1/2 cup heavy cream
- 2 teaspoons chicken bouillon
- 1 teaspoon dried basil
- 1/2 tsp EACH dried oregano, dried parsley
- 1/4 tsp EACH salt, pepper
- 3/4 cup freshly grated Parmesan cheese
- 1/3 cup shredded mozzarella cheese
- 2 cups roughly chopped spinach optional

Garnish

- freshly grated Parmesan cheese

INSTRUCTIONS

Chicken Rub

1. Whisk together seasonings listed under "Chicken" in a medium bowl. Drizzle then rub tops of chicken evenly with ½

tablespoon sun dried tomato olive oil then rub with half of Chicken Seasonings.

2. Flip chicken over and repeat using remaining Chicken Seasonings. Let rest while you prep the rest of the ingredients.

Pasta

1. Cook pasta al dente according to package directions in salted water.
2. Remove 1 cup pasta water before draining. Toss pasta with a drizzle of olive oil to keep it from sticking.
3. Set aside.

Cook Chicken

1. Heat 2 tablespoons sun-dried tomato olive oil in very large skillet with sides over medium high heat. Once very hot, add chicken and cook, undisturbed for 3-4 minutes, or until nicely browned on one side.
2. Turn chicken over, cover, and reduce heat to medium. Cook for approximately 3-5 more

minutes (depending on thickness of chicken), or until chicken is cooked through. Remove to a cutting board and tent with foil, do not clean out pan. Wait until ready to serve to slice or chop chicken.

Pasta Sauce

1. Melt 2 tablespoons butter in 1 tablespoon sun-dried tomato olive oil over medium-low heat in the same skillet.

2. Add sun-dried tomatoes and shallots and sauté 3-4 minutes, until shallots are tender, scraping up any brown bits left from chicken.

3. Add garlic and red pepper flakes (if using) and cook an additional 30 seconds. Sprinkle in flour and cook while stirring for 1 minute (it will be thick).

4. Turn heat to low then slowly whisk in chicken broth, milk, and heavy cream, stirring constantly until smooth. Stir in chicken bouillon and spices then increase

heat to medium high to bring sauce to a simmer. Simmer until thickened, stirring often. Reduce heat to low and stir in Parmesan cheese until melted, followed by mozzarella cheese until melted.

5. Stir in pasta until well coated followed by spinach. Add additional reserved pasta water a little at a time if needed to reach desired consistency.

6. Add sliced or chopped chicken and stir into pasta. Garnish with additional Parmesan if desired.

7. Taste and season with additional salt, pepper and/or red pepper flakes to taste. Garnish with freshly grated Parmesan Cheese and basil if desired.

CHEESY BROCCOLI, SAUSAGE, AND CAULIFLOWER CASSEROLE

INGREDIENTS

- 1 pound broccoli florets
- 1/2 pound cauliflower florets
- 1 tablespoon vegetable oil
- 1 small yellow onion, finely diced
- 3 cloves garlic, minced
- 12 ounces smoked sausage, polish or andouille, sliced into 1-inch rounds
- 8 ounces cream cheese, room temperature, cut into cubes for easier mixing
- 1/2 cup mayonnaise, or sub plain yogurt or sour cream
- 2 cups shredded mexican blend cheese, divided
- 2 tablespoons dijon mustard
- salt and fresh ground pepper, to taste

INSTRUCTIONS

1. Preheat oven to 400°F.
2. Lightly grease a 9x13 baking dish; set aside.
3. Add water to a large pot, filling it about halfway up, and bring to a boil.
4. Add broccoli florets and cauliflower florets to the boiling water.
5. Bring to a boil and continue to cook for 3 minutes. Drain well and set aside.
6. In the meantime, add vegetable oil to a skillet and heat over medium-high heat.
7. Stir in onions and cook for 2 minutes.
8. Add garlic and cook for 20 seconds.
9. Stir in smoked sausage and cook for 3 minutes, or until browned on all sides. Stir frequently.
10. Transfer broccoli, cauliflower, plus sausage mixture to previously prepared baking dish.
11. In a mixing bowl combine cream cheese, mayonnaise, 1 cup shredded cheese, dijon mustard, salt, and pepper; mix until thoroughly incorporated.

12. Stir the cream cheese mixture into the broccoli mixture; stir around until everything is well combined. Add remaining shredded cheese on top.

13. Bake for 12 to 15 minutes, or until cheese is melted and top is golden brown.

CHICKEN POTATO BAKE

INGREDIENTS

•4 medium potatoes, cut into ¾ inch/2 cm cubes (russet, white, and red are all good choices, no need to peel)

- •1 tablespoon minced garlic
- •1.5 tablespoons olive oil
- •⅛ teaspoon salt
- •⅛ teaspoon pepper
- •1.5 pounds boneless skinless chicken breasts or thighs (I like to use thighs)
- •¾ cup shredded mozzarella cheese
- •parsley (optional, freshly chopped)

INSTRUCTIONS

1. Preheat oven to 425 degrees F/220 degrees C.

2. Place the potato cubes in a large bowl, add the garlic, olive oil, salt, and pepper, and toss to coat.

3. 4 medium potatoes, cut into ¾ inch/2 cm cubes,1 tablespoon minced garlic,1.5 tablespoons olive oil,⅛ teaspoon salt,⅛ teaspoon pepper

4. Spray a large (9x13) baking dish with non stick spray. Spread potato mixture in dish and bake about 15 minutes.

5. Remove baking dish from oven and place the chicken pieces in the dish, nestling them down into the potato mixture a bit. If desired, brush the top of each chicken piece with a little olive oil and season with salt and pepper.

6. Bake 20-25 minutes, until chicken is cooked and potatoes are browned.

7. Sprinkle the mozzarella cheese over the top, return to the oven and bake for a few more minutes to melt the cheese.

8. When serving, sprinkle chopped parsley on top (if desired).

ROTISSERIE CHICKEN CASSEROLE

INGREDIENTS

- Meat from 1 Rotisserie Chicken shredded
- 3 cans of cream of chicken soup
- 3 Cups shredded Monterey Jack Cheese
- 3 Green Onions Cleaned and Chopped up
- Salt and Pepper
- ½ envelop of Hidden Valley Ranch powdered dressing mix dry
- 1 lb. of pre-cooked Bacon Crumbles or fry some up yourself – the pre-cooked just saves time.
- 1 lb. Fusilli pasta – squiggly kind

INSTRUCTIONS

1. Preheat the oven to 400F and set up two 9×9 pans or one 15×9 sprayed with non-stick spray.

2. Put shredded chicken into a big bowl or lay out on baking sheet and sprinkle with salt, pepper, and the HVR dry dressing mix then mix it up good and let it set.

3. Prepare pasta as directed then put pasta, cans of soup, 2 cups of cheese, onion, most all bacon, and the chicken.

4. Mix well – you will need a big pasta pot to do this in because that's a lot of food!

5. Using a ladle, dip the mixture into pan then sprinkle with bacon and finally the cheese.

6. Put into the oven and bake for 25 minutes or until the cheese has melted and started to turn brown.

7. Let it sit for about 10 minutes after you take it out and then serve with a salad!

CHICKEN LASAGNA

INGREDIENTS

- 12 lasagna noodles cooked and cooled
- 4 cups cooked chicken
- 3 cups vegetables cooked and cooled
- 10 oz frozen chopped spinach defrosted and squeezed dry
- 2 cups cottage cheese or ricotta cheese
- 2 eggs
- 2 tablespoons parsley
- 4 cups mozzarella divided
- ⅔ cup shredded parmesan cheese divided

Sauce

- ⅓ cup butter
- 1 onion diced
- 2 cloves garlic minced
- ¼ cup flour
- 2 cups milk
- 2 cups chicken broth
- 4 oz cream cheese

- 1 teaspoon dried basil
- ½ teaspoon oregano

INSTRUCTIONS

1. Preheat oven to 350°F.

Sauce

1. To make the sauce, melt butter, onion and garlic over medium low heat. Cook until onion is softened, about 3 minutes. Add flour and cook for 1-2 minutes.

2. Reduce heat to low. Combine milk and broth. Add a small amount at a time whisking to thicken. The mixture will become very thick, continue adding a little bit of liquid at a time whisking until smooth.

3. Once all of the liquid has been added, stir in cream cheese until melted.

4. Remove from heat and add in ⅓ cup parmesan, 1 cup mozzarella cheese, dried basil and oregano.

Assembly

1. Combine cottage cheese, eggs, parsley and spinach. Set aside.
2. In a 9x13 pan, layer 4 noodles, sauce, cooked vegetables and half of the chicken. Sprinkle with ½ mozza, ¼ cup parmesan and ⅓ of the sauce.
3. Add another layer of noodles, chicken, cottage cheese mixture, sauce. Top with noodles and sauce. Cover and bake 40 minutes.
4. Uncover, top with cheese and bake 20-30 minutes more.

ZUCCHINI MUSHROOM CHICKEN STIR FRY

INGREDIENTS

- 1 pound boneless skinless chicken breasts, cut into bite sized cubes (you can also use boneless, skinless chicken thighs)
- 2 tablespoons cornstarch

- 2 tablespoons vegetable oil
- 1 tablespoon minced garlic
- 1/2 tablespoon fresh minced ginger OR 1/2 teaspoon ground ginger
- 8 ounces white button mushrooms, sliced
- 1 zucchini, sliced into 1/4-INCH thick half moons
- 3 tablespoons gluten-free low-sodium soy sauce
- 1 tablespoon rice vinegar
- 2 teaspoons sugar
- sprinkle of toasted sesame seed oil, for garnish, optional
- sesame seeds, for garnish
- scallions, for garnish

INSTRUCTIONS

1. Place chicken pieces in a bowl and sprinkle with cornstarch; toss to coat.
2. Heat vegetable oil in a large skillet or a wok over medium-high heat; add chicken pieces to the hot oil and cook for 6 to 8 minutes, or

until browned on both sides and cooked through.

3. Remove chicken from wok or skillet and set aside.

4. Turn down heat to medium-low and add garlic and ginger to the skillet; cook and stir for 20 seconds, or just until fragrant.

5. Turn up the heat to medium-high and stir in the mushrooms and zucchini; cook for 4 minutes, or until fork tender and browned. Stir frequently.

6. In the meantime, in a small mixing bowl whisk together soy sauce, rice vinegar, and sugar.

7. Stir chicken back into the skillet.

8. Add in the prepared soy sauce and stir to coat chicken and veggies.

9. Stir and cook for 30 seconds to 1 minute, or until everything is heated through and sauce has slightly thickened.

10. Remove from heat; sprinkle with sesame oil and sesame seeds.

11. Garnish with scallions and serve.

SMOTHERED CHICKEN

INGREDIENTS

- 5 strips thick cut bacon
- 2 large boneless skinless chicken breasts
- 1/2 cup Vegetable oil, for frying.

Chicken Dredge

- 1/2 cup all-purpose flour
- ¼ cup breadcrumbs, plain or Italian
- 1 teaspoon seasoned salt
- ¾ teaspoon black pepper

Gravy

- 4 Tablespoons Butter
- 4 Tablespoons Flour
- 2.5 cups chicken broth
- 1 beef bouillon cube, or 1 tsp beef better than bouillon
- 1/3 cup half and half, (half milk, half cream)

- 1 teaspoon low sodium soy sauce, can sub Worcestershire sauce
- 1 teaspoon onion powder
- 1 teaspoon garlic powder
- ¼ teaspoon dried thyme
- ¼ teaspoon dried rosemary
- ¼ teaspoon ground sage
- 2-3 drops Kitchen Bouquet, optional

Instructions

1. Prework: Add chicken dredge ingredients to a large plate and toss to combine. Set aside. Measure out gravy ingredients prior to beginning.

2. Cook the Bacon: Fry bacon over medium-low heat until crispy on both sides. Remove from pan and pour grease into a heat-safe bowl. Reserve 2-4 Tablespoons of clear bacon drippings. Wipe any black residue from the pan if needed.

3. Slice & Pound the Chicken: While the bacon cooks, slice each chicken breast in half

lengthwise to create 2 thinner slices. Place saran wrap over them and use a meat tenderizer to pound them to about 3/4 inches thick. This gives them a little more texture for the flour dredge to hold on to. They'll plump up more when cooked.

4. Coat the Chicken: Wipe the chicken dry and coat generously in the flour mixture, get in every nook and cranny.

5. Cook the Chicken: Add the reserved bacon drippings to the clean pan and enough vegetable oil to cover the chicken by half. Heat over medium-high heat. Once heated and glistening, add the chicken. Fry 2 at a time for about 5 minutes per side, until they have a nice golden sear. Set aside on a plate. Adjust heat down slightly and back up throughout cooking as needed.

6. Drain the oil: Remove the oil from the pot and use a paper towel to remove any black spots from the pan, but leave any brown

remnants. This is called 'fond' and will give the gravy a nice flavor.

7. Make the Roux: Melt the butter over medium heat and use a silicone spatula to "clean" the bottom of the pan. Sprinkle the flour gradually, whisking continuously, until a paste forms.

8. Add the Broth and Half and Half: Add the liquid in small increments, whisking constantly. It will thicken up in between each splash of liquid. If you add it all at once, you'll "break" the roux and it won't be thick.

9. Add remaining gravy ingredients: Slowly add the beef bouillon, soy sauce, and seasonings.

10. Bring to a gentle boil, then reduce to a simmer. Add a few drops of kitchen bouquet if a darker color is desired.

11. Add the chicken back to the pan along with any juice from the plate.

12. Chop up the bacon and add it to the top of the chicken.

13. Cover partially and cook over low heat for 10-15 minutes. The internal temperature of the chicken should reach 165 degrees prior to serving.

14. Garnish with parsley and serve with mashed potatoes.

ZUCCHINI MUSHROOM CHICKEN STIR FRY

INGREDIENTS

- 1 pound boneless skinless chicken breasts, cut into bite sized cubes (you can also use boneless, skinless chicken thighs)
- 2 tablespoons cornstarch
- 2 tablespoons vegetable oil
- 1 tablespoon minced garlic
- 1/2 tablespoon fresh minced ginger OR 1/2 teaspoon ground ginger
- 8 ounces white button mushrooms, sliced

- 1 zucchini, sliced into 1/4-INCH thick half moons
- 3 tablespoons gluten-free low-sodium soy sauce
- 1 tablespoon rice vinegar
- 2 teaspoons sugar
- sprinkle of toasted sesame seed oil, for garnish, optional
- sesame seeds, for garnish
- scallions, for garnish

INSTRUCTIONS

1. Place chicken pieces in a bowl and sprinkle with cornstarch; toss to coat.
2. Heat vegetable oil in a large skillet or a wok over medium-high heat; add chicken pieces to the hot oil and cook for 6 to 8 minutes, or until browned on both sides and cooked through.
3. Remove chicken from wok or skillet and set aside.

4. Turn down heat to medium-low and add garlic and ginger to the skillet; cook and stir for 20 seconds, or just until fragrant.

5. Turn up the heat to medium-high and stir in the mushrooms and zucchini; cook for 4 minutes, or until fork tender and browned. Stir frequently.

6. In the meantime, in a small mixing bowl whisk together soy sauce, rice vinegar, and sugar.

7. Stir chicken back into the skillet.

8. Add in the prepared soy sauce and stir to coat chicken and veggies.

9. Stir and cook for 30 seconds to 1 minute, or until everything is heated through and sauce has slightly thickened.

10. Remove from heat; sprinkle with sesame oil and sesame seeds.

11. Garnish with scallions and serve.

CHICKEN POTATO BAKE

INGREDIENTS

•4 medium potatoes, cut into ¾ inch/2 cm cubes (russet, white, and red are all good choices, no need to peel)

•1 tablespoon minced garlic

•1.5 tablespoons olive oil

•⅛ teaspoon salt

•⅛ teaspoon pepper

•1.5 pounds boneless skinless chicken breasts or thighs (I like to use thighs)

•¾ cup shredded mozzarella cheese

•parsley (optional, freshly chopped)

INSTRUCTIONS

1. Preheat oven to 425 degrees F/220 degrees C.

2. Place the potato cubes in a large bowl, add the garlic, olive oil, salt, and pepper, and toss to coat.

3. 4 medium potatoes, cut into ¾ inch/2 cm cubes,1 tablespoon minced garlic,1.5 tablespoons olive oil,⅛ teaspoon salt,⅛ teaspoon pepper

4. Spray a large (9x13) baking dish with non stick spray. Spread potato mixture in dish and bake about 15 minutes.

5. Remove baking dish from oven and place the chicken pieces in the dish, nestling them down into the potato mixture a bit. If desired, brush the top of each chicken piece with a little olive oil and season with salt and pepper.

5.5 pounds boneless skinless chicken breasts or thighs

6. Bake 20-25 minutes, until chicken is cooked and potatoes are browned.

7. Sprinkle the mozzarella cheese over the top, return to the oven and bake for a few more minutes to melt the cheese.

8. ¾ cup shredded mozzarella cheese

9. When serving, sprinkle chopped parsley on top (if desired).

EASY BETTER-THAN-TAKEOUT SHRIMP FRIED RICE

INGREDIENTS:

- 2 tablespoons sesame oil
- 2 tablespoons canola or vegetable oil
- 1 pound medium-large fresh shrimp, cleaned (approximately 15-20 count shrimp)
- 1 cup frozen peas and diced carrots blend
- 1/2 cup corn (I use frozen straight from the freezer)
- 2 to 3 garlic cloves, finely minced or pressed
- 1/2 teaspoon ground ginger
- 3 large eggs, lightly beaten

- 4 cups cooked rice . To save time use two 8.8-ounce pouches cooked and ready-to-serve rice)
- 2 to 3 green onions, trimmed and sliced into thin rounds
- 3 to 4 tablespoons low-sodium soy sauce
- 1/2 teaspoon salt, or to taste
- 1/2 teaspoon freshly ground black pepper, or to taste

INSTRUCTIONS

1. To a large non-stick skillet or wok, add the oils, shrimp, and cook over medium-high heat for about 3 minutes, flipping halfway through. Cooking time will vary based on size of shrimp, don't overcook. Remove shrimp with a slotted spoon (allow oils and cooking juices to remain in skillet) and place shrimp on a plate; set aside.
2. Add the peas, carrots, corn, and cook for about 2 minutes, or until vegetables begin to soften, stir intermittently.

3. Add the garlic, ginger, and cook for 1 minute, stir intermittently.

4. Push vegetables to one side of the skillet, add the eggs to the other side, and cook to scramble, stirring as necessary.

5. Add the shrimp, rice, green onions, evenly drizzle with soy sauce, evenly season with salt and pepper, and stir to combine. Cook for about 2 minutes, or until shrimp is reheated through. Recipe is best warm and fresh but will keep airtight in the fridge for up to 5 days or in the freezer for up to 4 months. Reheat gently as desired.

ADRENAL FATIGUE DIET SMOOTHIE

INGREDIENTS

- 1 cup spinach
- ½ cup coconut water
- ½ orange (peeled)
- 1 cup pineapple (fresh or frozen)
- ½ cup cauliflower florets (frozen)

- 1 tablespoon fresh turmeric (or 1 teaspoon ground turmeric)
- 1 tablespoon flaxseed oil
- adaptogenic herbs (optional]
- 1 serving Protein Smoothie Boost (optional (

INSTRUCTIONS

1. Blend spinach, coconut water, and orange in blender until smooth.
2. Add remaining ingredients and blend until smooth.
3. Pour into a glass and enjoy!

Printed in Great Britain
by Amazon

40841973R00057